Heavenly Creation

Meditation for Care Givers

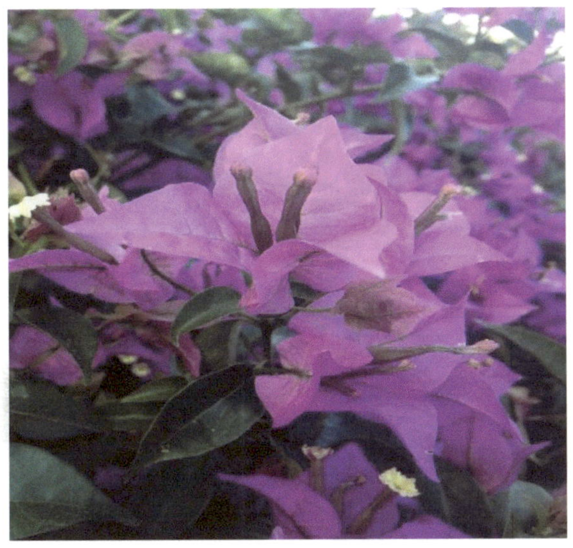

Frances Stroh RN, Ph.D., FCN

Photography by Joseph R. Reed

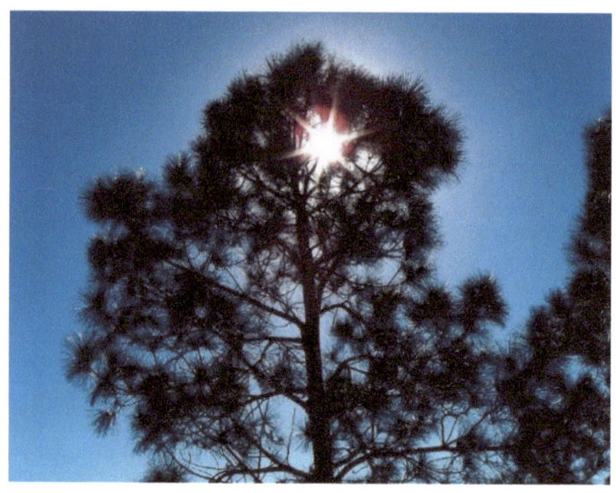

Touch of Life Care

Established in 1991

Caring, Counseling, Education, Information

http://www.tolcare.com

http://www.franstroh.com

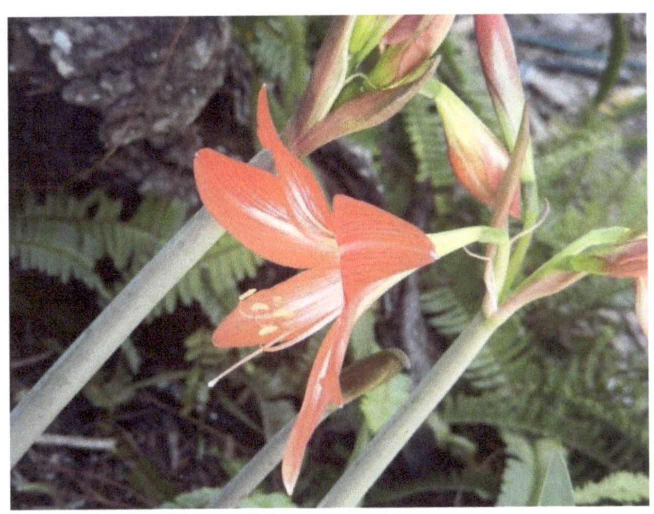

Dedication and Appreciation

Joseph R. Reed, Thank you and appreciation, always, for your berautiful, inspirational photography, and expert technical support.

Dedication and thank you to God, my Angels, my husband, family, friends, all my children and grandchildren..

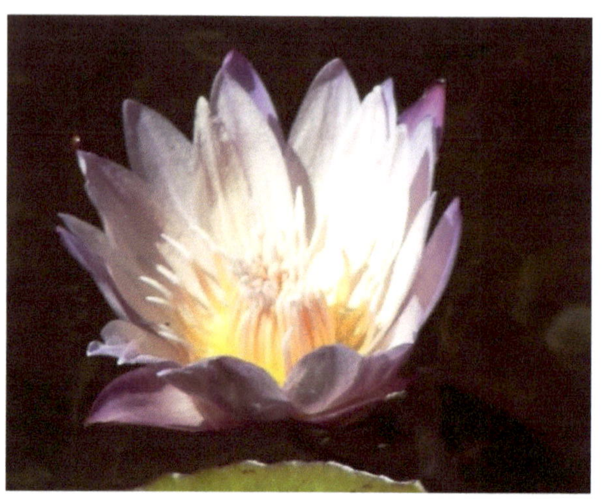

Introduction

Peace and comfort of our mind, body, and spirit is a Divine Creation and Gift of God. Everything is a form of perfection with the purpose of eternal life, inner peace and health. This book contains devotions for supporting a peaceful mind through increased awareness of our Spiritual connection with the Creator. Unconditional love and compassionate consideration promotes healing. We are guided to understand, give, and accept unconditional love that will bring sanctity to the soul and inner healing. This is accomplished through cognitive and meditative methods of care. The inner mind is connected with the mind of the Creator God. The beauty and wonders of creation are captured in photographic imagery and meditative prayer. Each meditation promotes a sense of inner peace for healing.

Table of Contents

Introduction 3

Meditation for Abiding Peace 6

The True Healer 7

Sacred Unity 8

Living in the Light 9

Living in a Spiritual World 10

Our Spiritual Nature 11

The Nature of Miracles 12

Laws of Nature 13

Move into Holy Light 14

Spiritual Care 15

Imagery for Health 16

Talking to God in Prayer 17

God Lives 18

Healing Light of God 19

Spirit of the Lord God 20

God is Everywhere 21

Our Divine Nature 22

Enter the Kingdom of God 23

Philosophy of Consciousness 24

Inspired Living 25

Divine Trust 26

Awareness of Guiding Light 27

Divine Light and Love 28

Light in the Darkness 29

The Way of Peace.. 30

Divine Healing.. 31

Rest in the Holy Spirit 32

Love Unconditionally.. 33

Inner Reflection 34

Shelter in Divine Spirit 35

Secure in the Peace of God 36

Spiritual Growth 37

Prayer for Holy Guidance 38

The Spirit of God 39

Sacred Love 40

Awaken to the Holy Light 41

Enlighten Your Mind... 42

Reference... 43

About the Author 44

Meditation for Abiding Peace

Within your mind, pray and request guidance from God. Only good, helpful, thoughts, and feelings will influence you in any way. Mentally surround yourself with a shield of the Holy Spirit. You are in total control and influenced only by feelings of joy and comfort as you enter a state of meditative prayer. Relax each muscle of your body and quiet your thoughts in silent meditation for a few moments. Focus and clear your mind. Breathe in deeply and exhale slowly. Imagine the air filling with a heavenly scent of fragrant flowers. With each breath, become more peaceful and calmer. Imagine a journey to a beautiful location of serenity and comfort in the Holy Presence of God. Move gently forward as though you are floating peacefully toward your destination. You can see from a distance that sacred and Holy Place where you are completely protected and secure.

Now visualize yourself moving toward this location of complete peace and contentment. Your path is glowing with Holy Light. It is so pleasant in this atmosphere of serenity. Just continue to become more relaxed, as you rest and be at peace. Your sense of serenity increases as you continue. Receive this guidance and Holy Blessings. Image yourself filled, surrounded, and protected by the Healing Light of God. Sacred Holy Spirit is helping you to resolve any problem. You may return to this location in the Presence of God at any time by just becoming aware of this Holy Light entering your mind and body. You are a blessed creation and child of God. Rest there for a few moments in silence. Let your mind remain quiet as you receive Divine inspiration for healing.

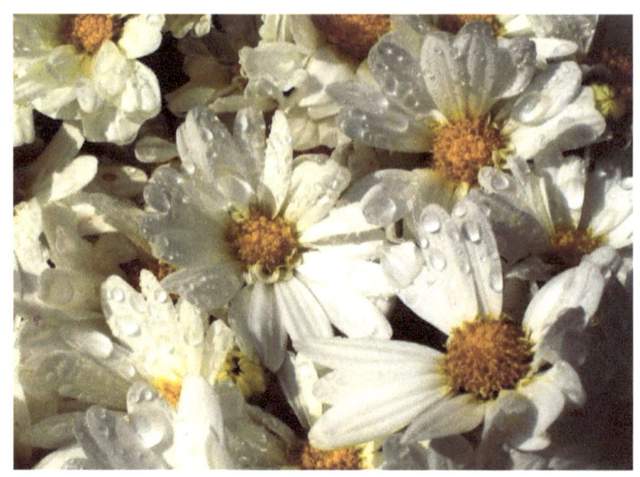

The True Healer

Spiritual Healing indicates that God or a power and intelligence that is beyond and greater than our self is the healer. We live by faith, which is to believe without knowing. Therefore, the purpose of spiritual care is to include our greatest healer which is faith, hope, and love. The Creator, God, is the true healer. Think of each person a being someone that you truly love and treat them accordingly. This is my mother, father, sister, brother, the one that I love in Divine Spirit. As we do for the one that we love, we do for all. The True Healer is the Love of God that we share with each other.

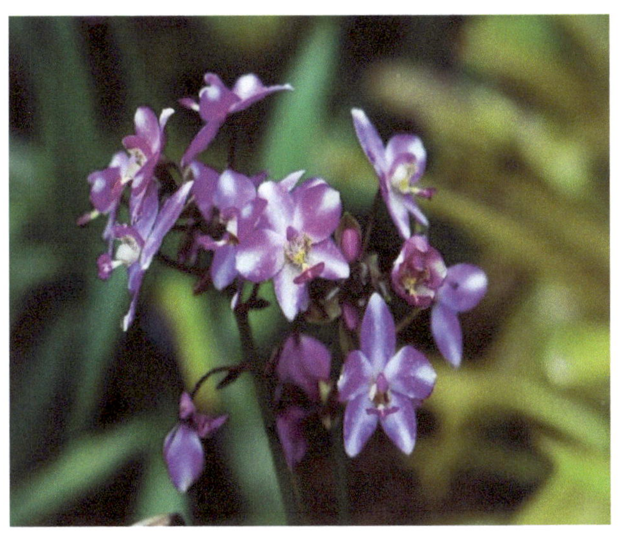

Sacred Unity

Spiritual Healing is an art and science that leads to wholeness and wellbeing. It provides care for the whole person, alleviates pain, and brings comfort. This leads to a sense of Sacred unity that is healing for the mind, body, and soul. We are providing care for a "human energy field disturbance." that includes the whole person and leads to comfort and relief of pain. Prescribe for each person, love, kindness, empathy and compassion. This is our Beloved Friend in the Divine Spirit of Sacred Unity.

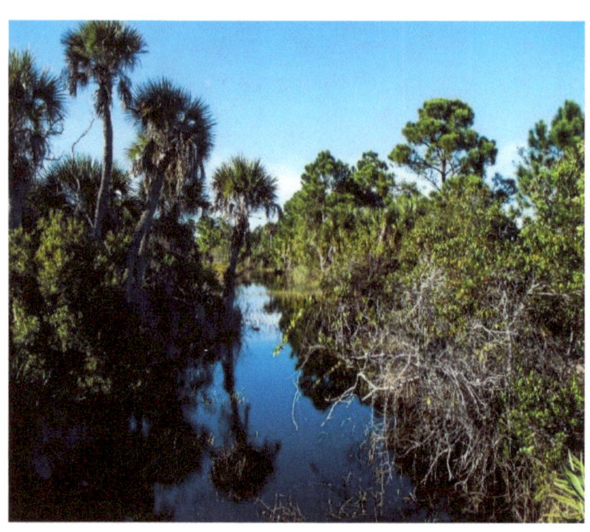

Living in the Light

We do not know what the mind is and how it works or everything that it is capable of accomplishing. But we do know that the mind has its own ways of causing what we imagine by bringing about responses in our physical bodies. Using creative visualization, the mind has the capability of healing any condition. This includes using the process of positive affirmation which is highly effective. See only good, hear only good, speak only good. Darkness and adversity are eliminated and vanquished in the Light. Live in the Light and be a light worker for the Creator.

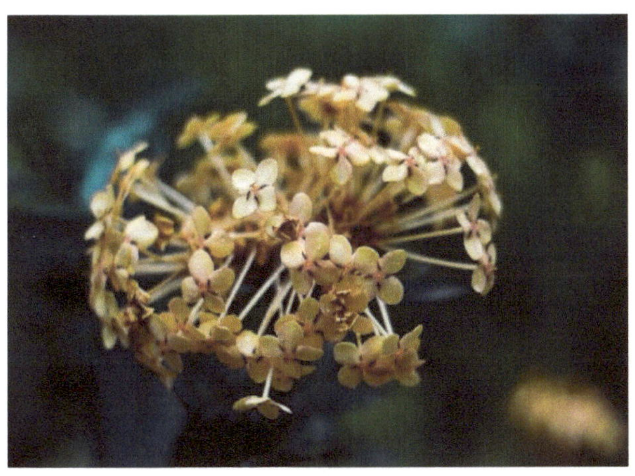

Living in a Spiritual World

We know that the mind controls our feelings and perceptions. There are multiple cases of spiritual healing. The reality is that everything including physical objects, when broken down to a state of the smallest known substance, is energy, which is Spirit. Our mind is part of the Universal Mind of God. The mind works like a computer that stores all information and memory. Our Mind is the controller of our life, feelings, and health. Our thoughts create our reality and feeling. We are living in a Spiritual World. Think pleasant, and uplifting thoughts and extend them to all who you know and love.

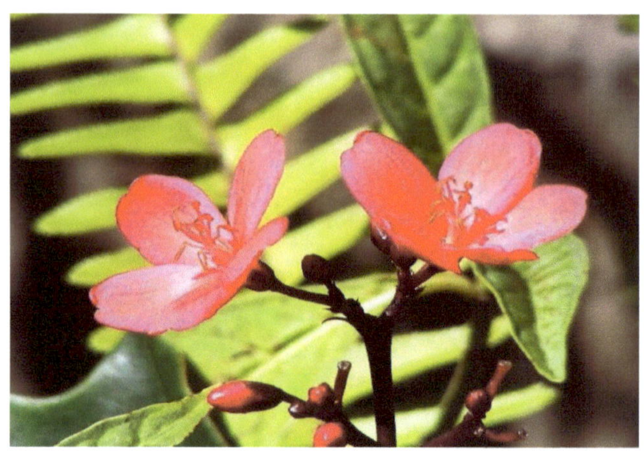

Our Spiritual Nature

Everyone is spiritual. Spirituality is natural for all people; it is the individual conscious self becoming aware that we are more than a physical being. We are composed of mind, body, and spirit. The spiritual self has immense ability. Healing of the Spirit leads to healing of the body. It is called the higher self, higher power, or consciousness. The name is not needed, just the consciousness of being connected in a spirit of love and caring for yourself and others. Become aware of your Spiritual Nature. Know yourself and you know the existence of a greater healing reality within the Divine Mind.

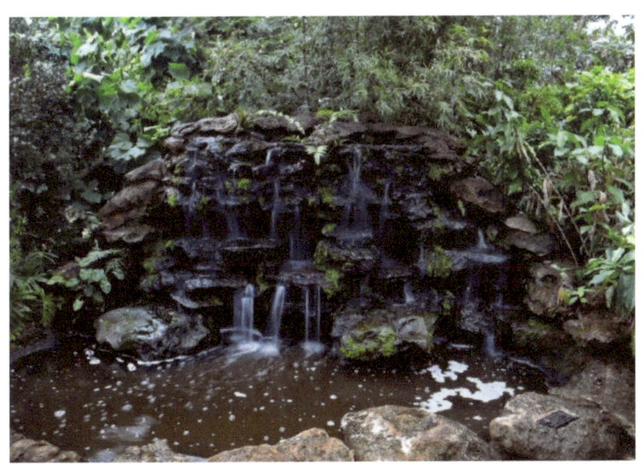

The Nature of Miracles

A miracle is an event that is unexplainable. Wherever there is life, the laws of God are at work. An injury is repaired by the laws which God created. Everything is the result of Divine Intelligence. There is a natural Divine rule that is restorative. Natural miracles occur every day. Belief in the natural laws make it ordinary. When we believe that God performed a miracle, amazingly it becomes supernatural. Creation, and all that we are and see, is the Nature of true miracles. Everything is created from nothing. The awesome miracle is that we have the power to recreate according to our gift of free will.

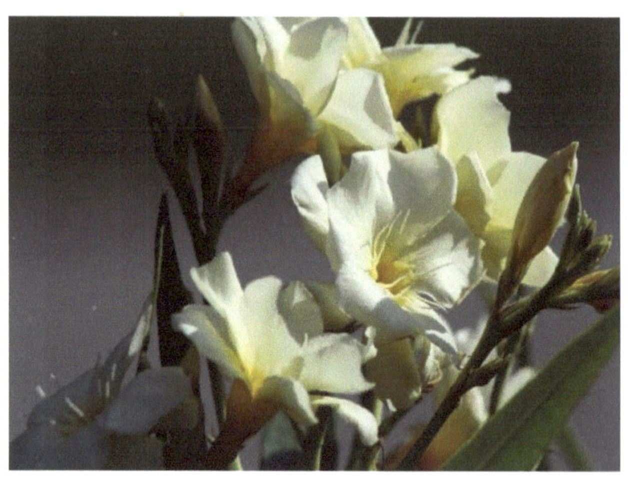

Laws of Nature

There are natural directives that govern everything in the universe including our bodies. In the beginning, God created the Heavens and the Earth with order, harmony, and intelligence. We are created to be well and healthy. Illness is the result when a Divine Law is violated. To remain healthy, we must cooperate with that same principle and create natural miracles. Live by the Law of Divine Unconditional Love for health, healing, and inner peace. Faith and Trust are healers of our Soul, by the Grace of God who created the Laws of Nature.

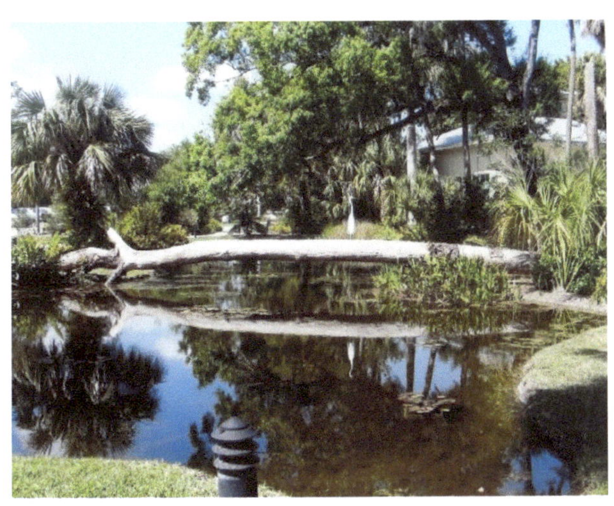

Move into Holy Light

It is impossible within the earth to be perfectly good. God knows this, God loves us always, and forgives. The law is so complex and detailed that the human soul, without Divine Grace and intervention, is lost in this world of spiritual darkness. Prayer and meditation lead us into the Holy Light. There is a spiritual world within the hidden levels of consciousness where we find heaven. Existence in this realm depends upon our belief. We have the freedom to become conscious of the true reality . Move forward into the Holy Light and return to guide others.

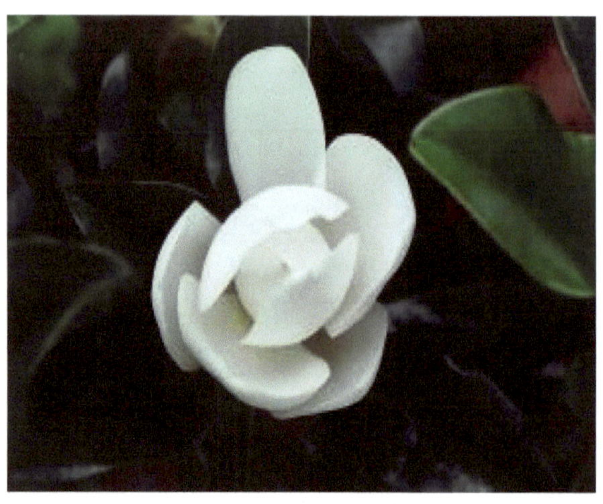

Spiritual Care

In a situation that is stressful, learn effective and individual methods of dealing with these events God's Way. Talk to God in prayer. Ask for guidance and help in each situation. Always do what is right according to God's Will and devise a plan of action accordingly. It is important to take into consideration the physical, emotional, and mental factors. Use effective methods of self-regulation by learning healthy strategies for dealing with problems and changes. Learn to adapt to each situation that arises by having faith and trust that God is in charge and taking care of you and all whom you love.

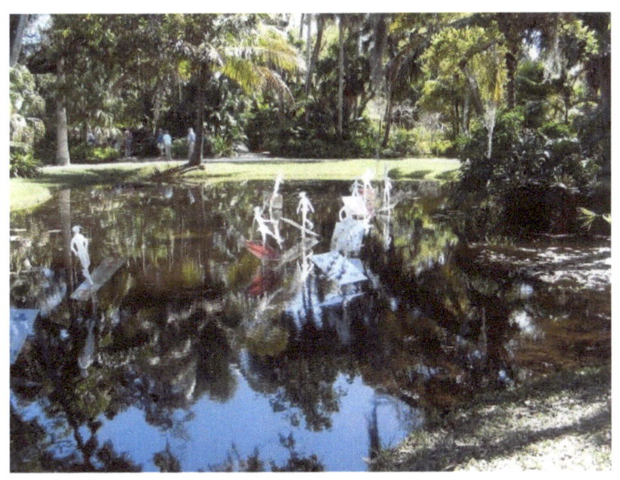

Imagery for Health

Imagery includes effective breathing and relaxation techniques. Helpful suggestion leads to constructive change. Imagery induces a very peaceful state of relaxation. It alleviates pain and promotes comfort. Your natural healing response is stimulated leading to improved health and faster healing during illness. Healthy individuals practice imagery to promote and maintain health. You create your reality within the mind. Think good, pleasant thoughts. Image your perfect reality and cause it to happen. You are the builder of your world and the master of your thoughts and feelings.

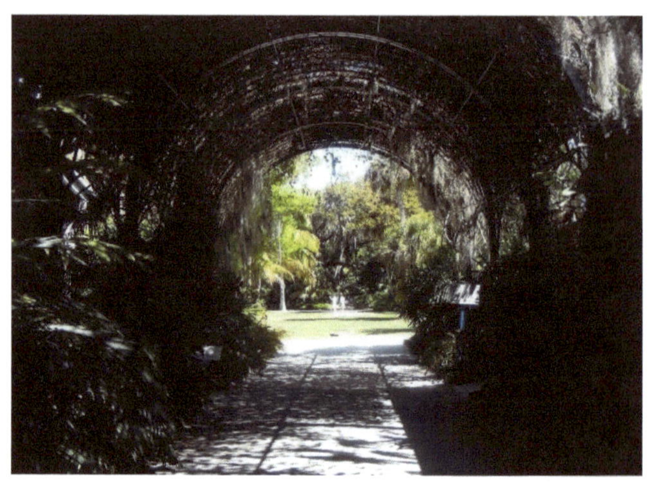

Talking to God in Prayer

Prayer is talking to God. Meditation is silently waiting and listening for guidance through Divine inspiration. The response flows from a place of Divine Intelligence, Wisdom, and Truth. An elevation in spiritual awareness, ultimate peace, and mental calmness is the result. There is a healing effect on the body, mind and spirit. It is the ability to direct attention to a place of silence and peace where you are in harmony with the Creator. We learn to direct thoughts away from worry and remain in the present moment. Inner guidance, heightened awareness, and a higher level of consciousness occur.

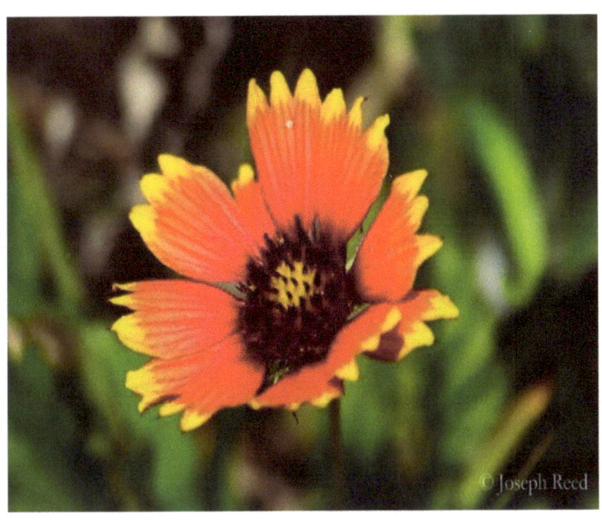

God Lives

Rest now and pray. Let the Holy Spirit of God be your Guide. Imagine yourself in the sacred presence of God. Feel the presence of peace, love, and holiness. God lives with and within us. Healing of body, mind, and soul is through communication with the mind of God. Our purpose is elevation of the consciousness through the Divine Spirit within us. This is accomplished through meditative prayer. I believe, but only God knows. The interpretation of the term "I Am" is that I Am all that there is, I Am everything. I Am the eternal presence. God is One, and for all people.

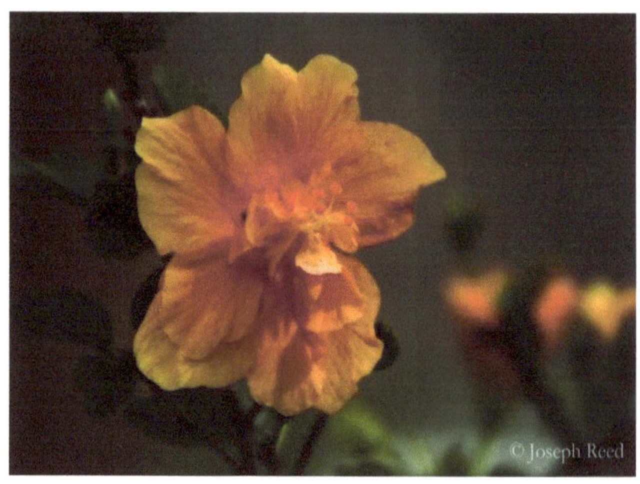

Healing Light of God

The Light of God shines into our life, as we pray and meditate. Our mission is to bring inner peace and healing love to those in need. Difficulties begin within our own mind and are resolved as we pray. Healing the sick is a gift of the Holy Spirit. We pray for Sacred Light in this place of darkness. Only Divine Power heals. This gift is given to all who ask with sincere belief, faith, love and compassion. Help us to understand and to believe that only goodness is of You. We thank You God for all your Blessings.

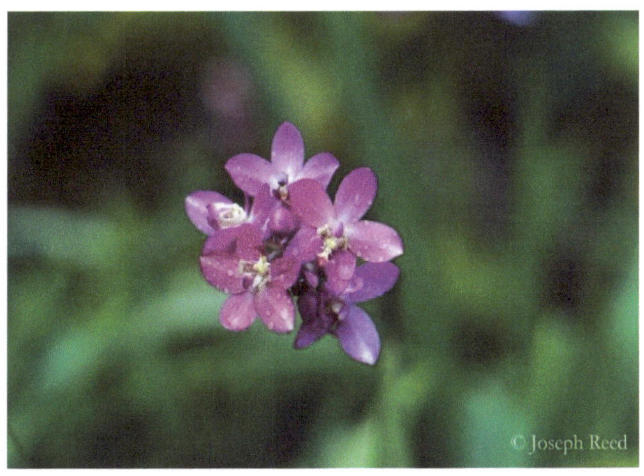

Spirit of the Lord God

It is the Will of God, that we have unconditional love for all. Accept all of God's creation, as part of one whole and complete picture. There are various methods of expressing feelings, thoughts and beliefs. The Spirit of God manifests in many forms, but is always the same, eternal, everywhere and in everything. The Spirit of the Lord God is upon us all. We have a mission to bring God's word to the afflicted, to heal the broken hearted, and to bring freedom to those who are captive to illness and adversity.

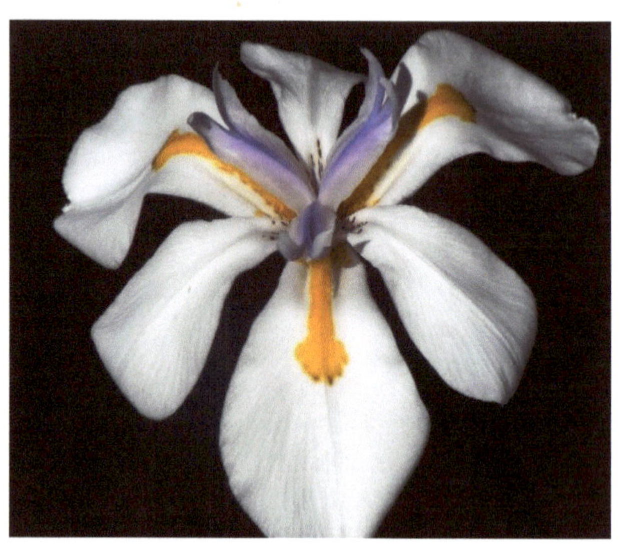

God is Everywhere

God is living here and now in every move and every breath. God is life and Love. God is all things, all creation. We live and move in the Spirit of God. God is the energy of life and the way that leads us, motivates us, and gives us our being. Reality is the manifestation of an object that we see, hear, feel, and believe. We have eyes, so we can see, and we have ears to hear. Look and listen, God is everywhere and in all things. God is life and the life that is in all things and all of existence.

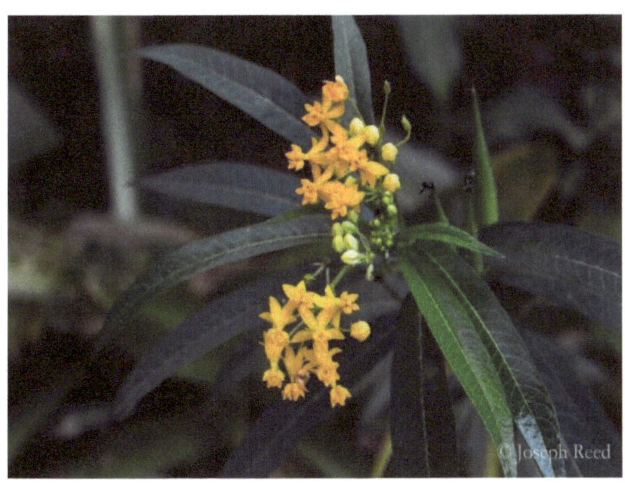

Our Divine Nature

The living God is of us. God exists, moves, and has being in every living thing. God is eternal, and always present. God is life. God is everything. There is matter, which is physical, has substance and occupies space. This is very real. There is energy which makes things move and have life. This is very real. We have intelligence, emotion, and feeling. All these things exist here and now and are part of all living beings. All that we experience is an expression of the Divine nature of our Creator who is only good.

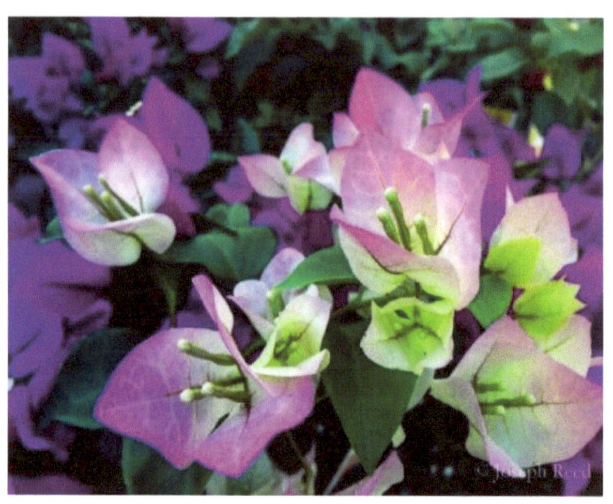

Enter the Kingdom of God

God is beyond our ability to understand, beyond science, and unreachable through thought but ever present in eternal sacred spirit. This is where we find the solution to problems. We can reevaluate events from a more advanced and mature perspective to heal and release inner conflict. Awareness of higher dimensions exists within the mind where everything is a possibility. Enter this realm with a spirit of love and compassion. Internal images are derived from a limitless, collective mind. Control is always in accord with our own belief. Become aware of each blessing.

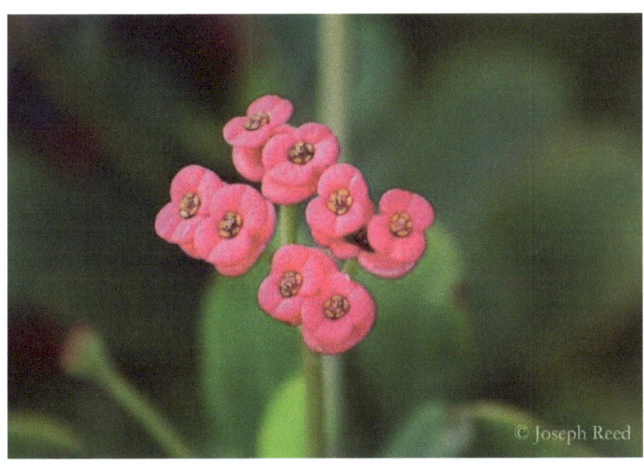

Philosophy of Consciousness

The philosophy of consciousness reveals that everything is consciousness and that our reality is created within the mind. Scientific theory related to quantum physics explains how it is scientifically possible to influence physical matter with the mind and our thoughts. This is important to understand since it is necessary to believe and have faith for healing to occur. Divine consciousness is the mind of God working in our life. This is a mind that is beyond our understanding but knows all things. We have a sacred nature and relate to the Mind of God.

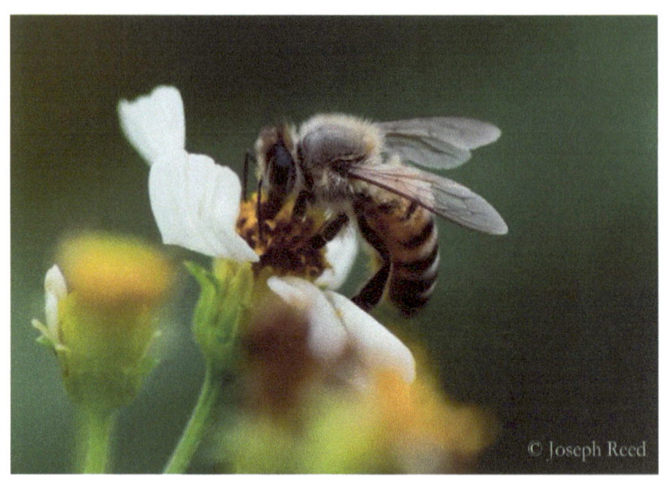

Inspired Living

Dear Lord God, surround and protect us, as we enter Your Sacred Place of peace, goodness, and love. Guide us on this path of spiritual growth and bring us closer to you. Our Lord God, we ask You to always be our guide. As we open our mind and heart, help us to listen, so that we hear your voice, and let your word flow into our thoughts and spirit. Fill us with your Holy Spirit, and let the Light of Your Sacred love, peace and healing enter our mind, heart, soul and life. Bless us, and all for whom we pray. Give us faith to believe that all who we know, and love, are safely in your care. Bless us with your gift of grace and faith,

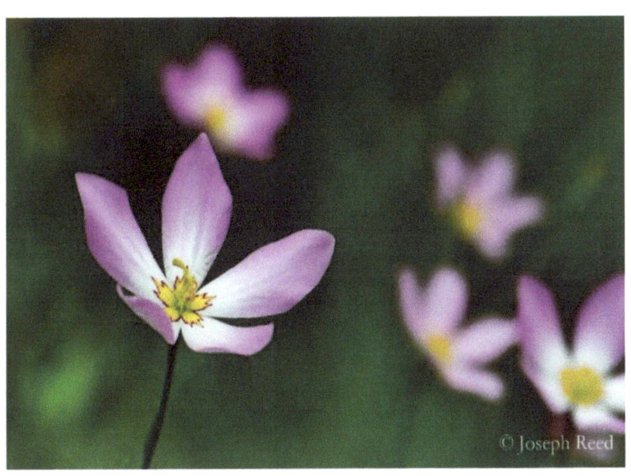

Divine Trust

Trust, that God is caring for everything and everyone. This is the way to true peace. Meditation leads to a quiet mind and focus on the present moment. Our inner mind is then prepared to resolve any problem. Divine time is here and now, and it is eternity. Inner guidance flows from Sacred Holy Presence. Only good is from God. Darkness can never exist in the Light of God. Accept only peaceful, loving thoughts and feelings. Always be aware. Immediately change any uncomfortable thought or feeling. Pray, Light of God, Spirit of God, be my guide. Let only Your Sacred Peace and Love influence me in any way.

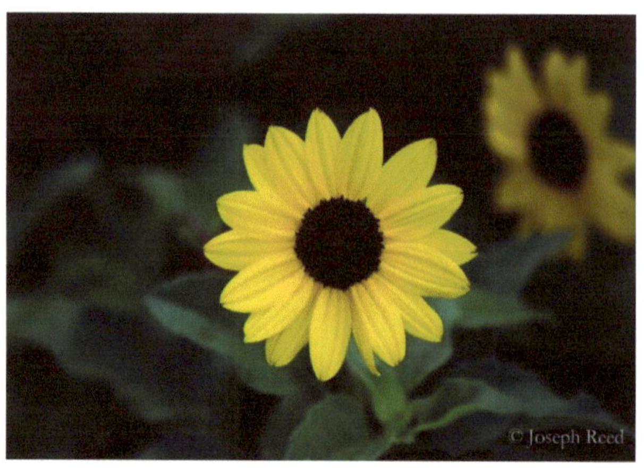

Awareness of Guiding Light

Lord God fill us with Your Holy Spirit of wisdom and truth. Guide our mind, heart and soul. Help us to be truly discerning as we receive inspiration and guidance. Allow only Your Holy Spirit to be of any influence during this meditation and always. Lead us closer to Your Divine Presence. Help us to listen and understand our purpose in this life. Reveal Divine Sacred truth and fill our mind, heart, and soul with your loving peace and Holy Presence. Be our shelter and protector during this time of prayer and always. We rest now, in Divine loving care. Our awareness of Sacred Guiding Light is increasing, as it flows peacefully.

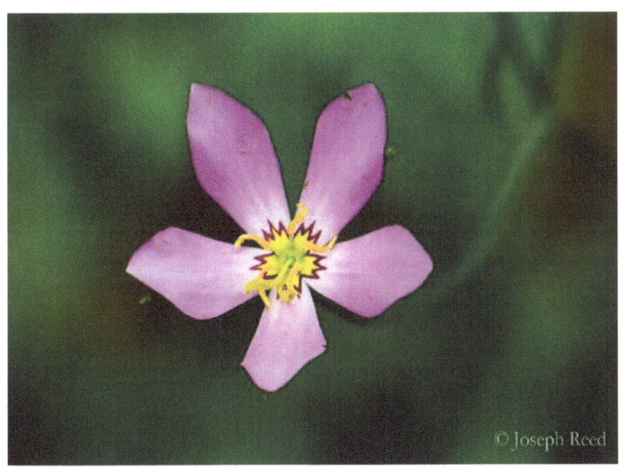

Divine Light and Love

With each breath, become more serene and content. Now breathe in, exhaling slowly, feeling calm, at ease, flowing, at peace. You can continue now breathing easily and become more peaceful. Your mind is clear and receptive. It is like a calm lake receiving replenishment from a flowing stream, ready to experience and enjoy new things, ready to understand. You are at ease feeling good. Continue to relax more peacefully. Breathe easily and freely. You are becoming more peaceful, comfortable and at ease with each breath. The Holy Light of God surrounds and always protects you.

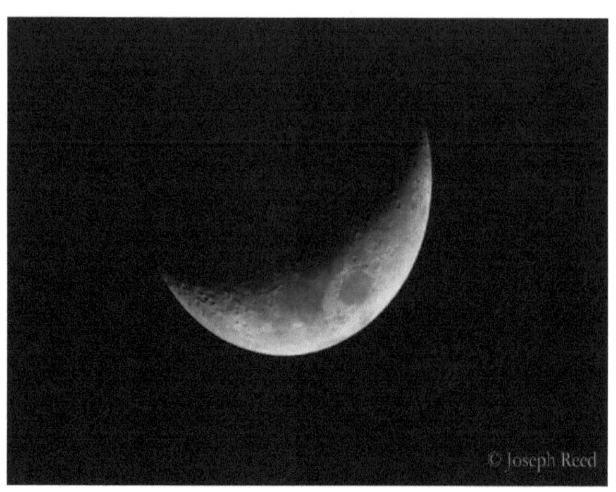

Light in the Darkness

There is a gentle soothing flow throughout our being, as we receive compassionate and loving spiritual care. As we receive, we learn to give. It is like waves in an ocean of warm fluid that projects love and protection merging all into one. In this bonding, we are in touch with the Holy Presence of God. There is knowledge and wisdom, giving meaning to life. It is an awakening from a dream, in which all was vague and meaningless, and now the reality of life is apparent, and we feel wonderful. As we know what we need, we know how to extend love and compassion to others in a peaceful and comforting way.

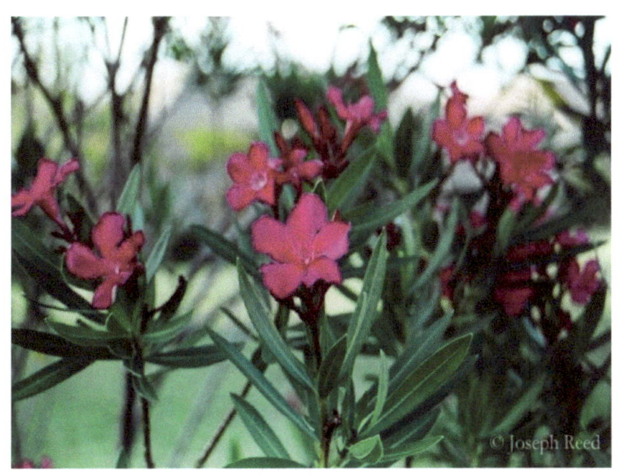

The Way of Peace

Think only good thoughts, see only good, hear only good, and speak only good. This is the way to inner peace and healing. Miracles then occur, leading to total healing of body, mind, and soul. You are well and healthy. This is the Divine Scheme and purpose of life. Belief, prayer, and faith are the way to God. Change your mind, attitude, abilities, and circumstances in a way that leads to mental peace. You are feeling peaceful and joyful. Your inner mind is working to resolve any problem through God's Holy Spirit. In this place we have the power to accomplish all in a perfect way according to the Will of God.

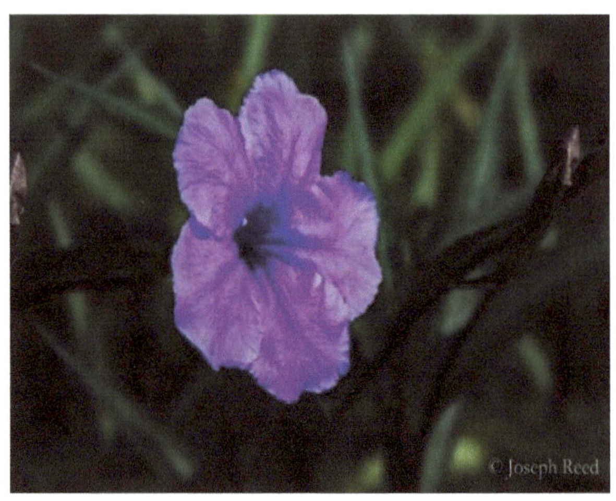

Divine Healing

You are in a pleasant, peaceful place where you can express your feelings with confidence. God is kind, understanding, and our true friend. This is where we solve a problem, heal an illness, or any situation that is influencing our life now. Take a moment to clarify your thoughts and then speak to God within your mind. As you rest your mind, release any problem or situation to God. Within your mind and with the grace of God, you have the power to direct yourself and your life. You are peaceful and in total control. God forgives any error and you can renew each situation that arises in God's perfect way.

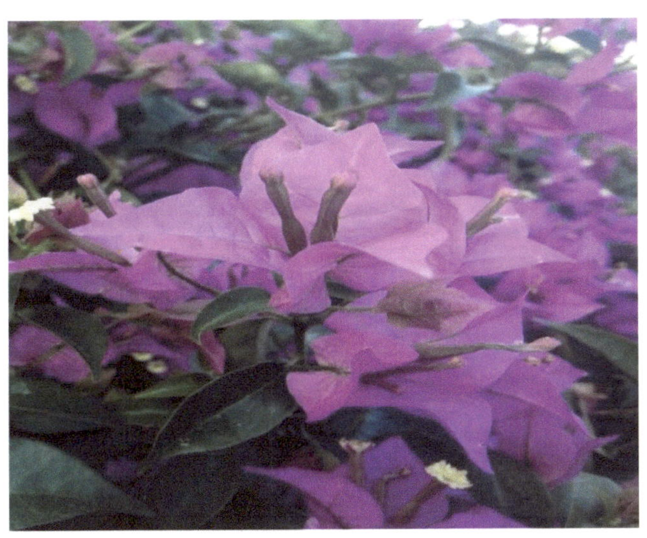

Rest in the Holy Spirit

Rest and pray. Holy Spirit of God protect and guide us as we pray and meditate. Fill us with your Love and bring us closer to you. Breathe in deeply and exhale slowly. As you exhale, begin to become aware of a sensation of absolute peace. Clear your mind of all thought for a moment. You are entering a place of unlimited awareness in the Holy Presence of God. Become aware that all is perfect and beautiful. All is good. God is only good. You are secure and sense a feeling of inner strength and comfort that flows from the Holy Spirit.

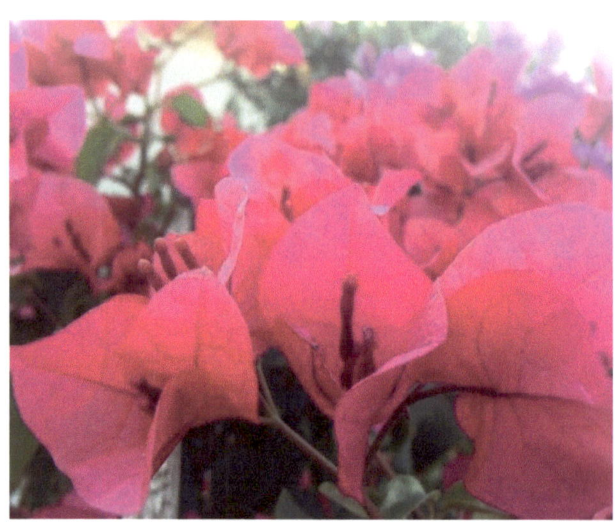

Love Unconditionally

Loving God be with us now. Help us to be loving and kind, even in times of trial. Teach us to forgive, and to love unconditionally. Forgive us any transgression, whether known or unknown. We sincerely pray for Unity, between all people. If all were sensitive and understanding of the rights and beliefs of others. It would be on earth as it is in Heaven, where there is only perfect health and joy. Faith, the power of prayer, and quiet meditation, enlightens our mind, leading to Inner Peace and Unity. Help us to experience true understanding of Oneness in Your Holy Spirit.

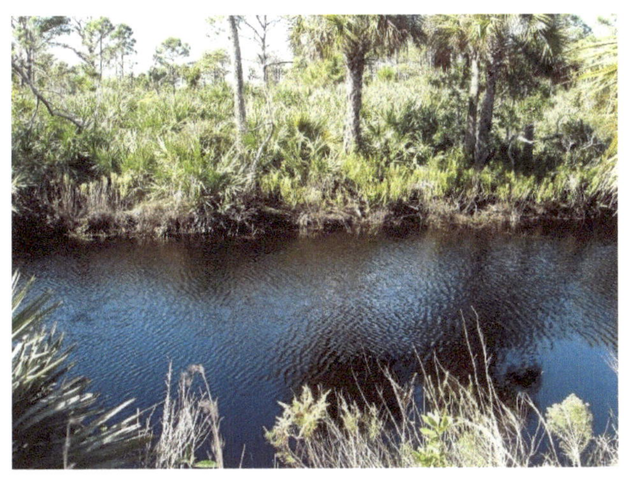

Inner Reflection

God is always waiting to help and to guide us. There is a sanctuary, within us, where we find inner peace. This is our entrance to a sacred place of peace. Through Divine Guidance, we enter using our natural ability to create within the mind. There is an expanded response to images and inspiration. We are always in control. Awareness is increased leading to foresight and understanding. Our mind is more attentive and discerning of circumstances. Understanding beyond the ordinary transpires. We can renew beliefs that change our concept of living, as we reflect inward and image God's flawless existence.

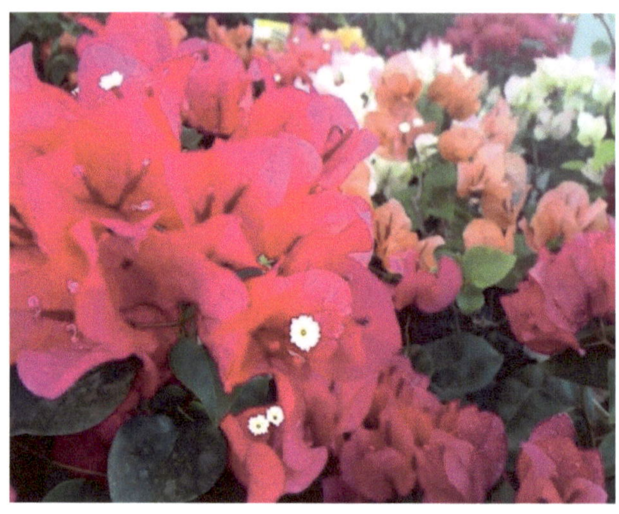

Shelter in Divine Spirit

Image yourself feeling secure and protected in a shelter of healing Divine Light. Holy Spirit protects and cares for you always. Rest your mind and transform any thought that enters your mind into peaceful harmony according to Sacred Holy Will. Breathe in deeply. Breathe out and let the air move gently, causing a flow of relaxation throughout your body. Now continue to breathe normally. You are resting in the shelter of God's Holy Spirit. God is with you, around you, and at your side, now and eternally.

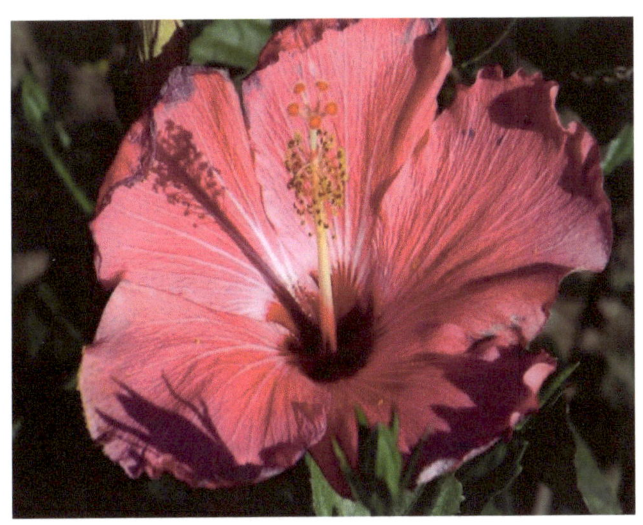

Secure in the Peace of God

Imagine that you are reflecting radiant Holy Light. Rest, and renew your mind and soul in the Spirit of God. Enter a special place where you are peaceful and secure. Sense the presence of Blessed Love. As you view from a distance, a Light appears and fills the surrounding area. This Light is surrounding you, protecting, purifying and relaxing your mind, body, and soul. This is the Healing Light of God. Protecting, Guiding, and Enlightening. You are Secure in the Peace of God, Now and Eternally.

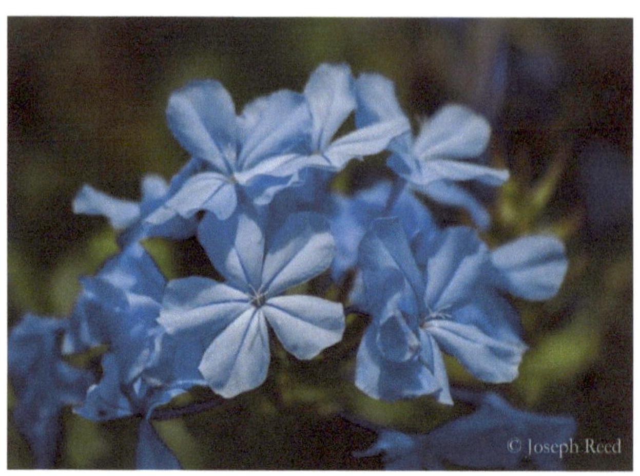

Spiritual Growth

A Sacred design for your life is apparent. The spiritual growth of your soul is steady and planned by the Grace of God. You are a creation of love and beauty formed in the image, spirit, and breath of the Creator. There is consciousness of yourself as a unique and perfect being. There is awareness of life and understanding that it is precious. Become one in Eternal Spirit. There is comfort of the soul and rest for your mind in the Love of God. This is the true reality that leads to spiritual growth, inner healing and heavenly peace.

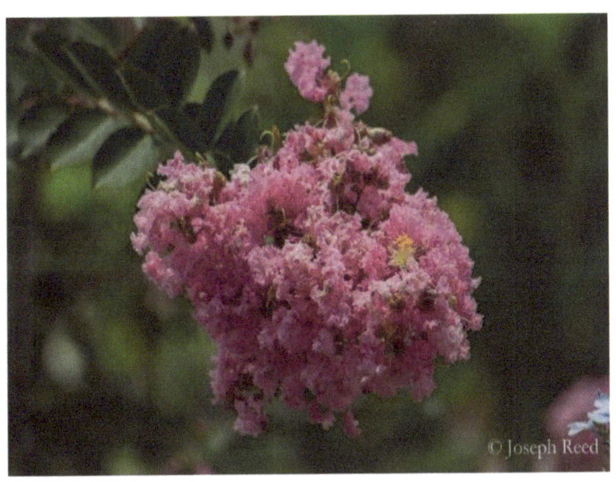

Prayer for Holy Guidance

Dear God, help us to receive Holy Guidance, as we pray and meditate. Guide our thoughts and bring deeper meaning and fulfillment to our life. Help us, that we may be of greater service to all who are in need. Help us to think always of goodness, and love. Guide us to speak words of strength, caring, and compassion. Strengthen our belief and faith. Help us to love and always show kindness to those around us, knowing that this will be of comfort to all. Bring blessings into our life, and the lives of all who we know and love. Bless us with Your Grace, that we may know the Truth.

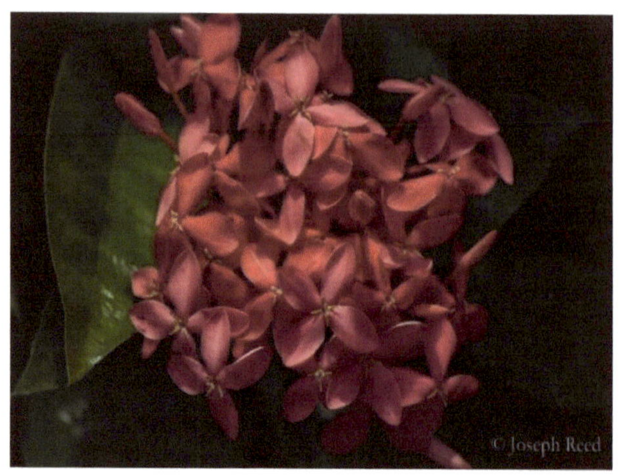

The Spirit of God

God is living and visible in all of life and nature. Life is so intricate and detailed, that intelligent purpose is undeniable. God lives in all that is Life. God is Energy, Spirit, the Light, that gives reason for all of existence. God is the perfection and detail of every phase of being. This is a deep mystery that we do not comprehend, but must experience, as we feel the presence of Love. The Stillness of the Mind during silent contemplation leads to a vision of Heaven on Earth. God is Universal, Eternal, Creative Energy, the Light, permeating and filling all with Life.

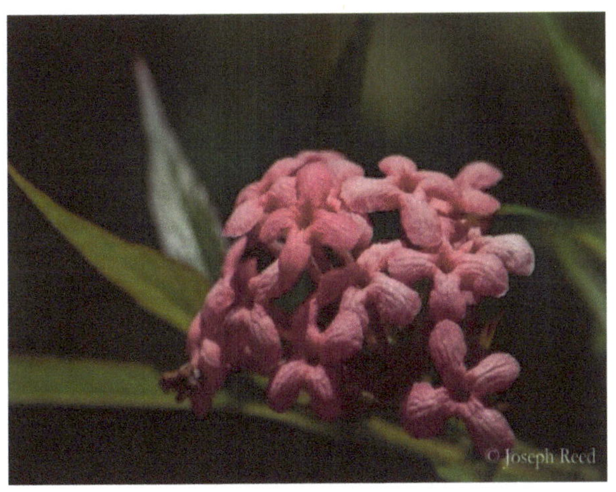

Sacred Love

Pray, and rest. Focus on a Holy mission and accomplish all tasks in God's perfect way, and according to Divine Will. Live in the moment, as we extend empathetic understanding, and care toward others. Listen, and respond, with care and consideration. We receive in return, that which we send out. Every moment, that we are aware of Holy Will we are living life in harmony and with an awareness of Divine Perfection. Healing love is filling our life, as we extend healing and love to all. Become aware of the feeling of Love. Completely relax your mind and body, and accept the flow of Sacred Love, that is with you now and always.

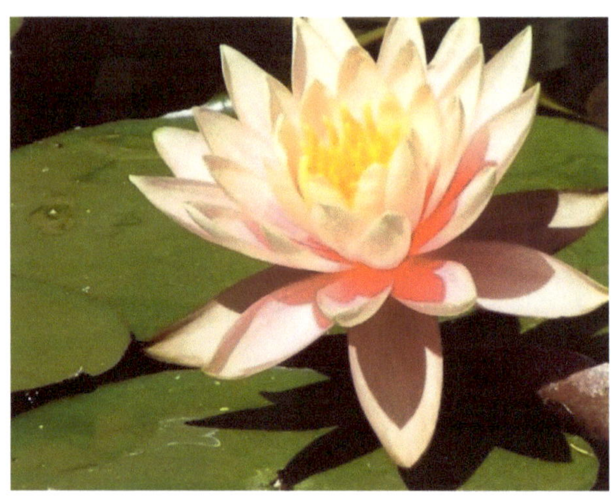

Awaken to the Holy Light

You are renewed, refreshed, and vital in this scheme of living. You can sense and feel life and love. Eternal mind, spirit, and matter are joining in a design for fulfillment. Connect now in an Eternal bond, which fills your life with blessed peace and comfort. Magnify and see with clarity each new being, flower, tree and all forms of life. You are a child of God. You are a child of Goodness. The Breath for Life Eternal fills your soul as you awaken in the light of this perfect day.

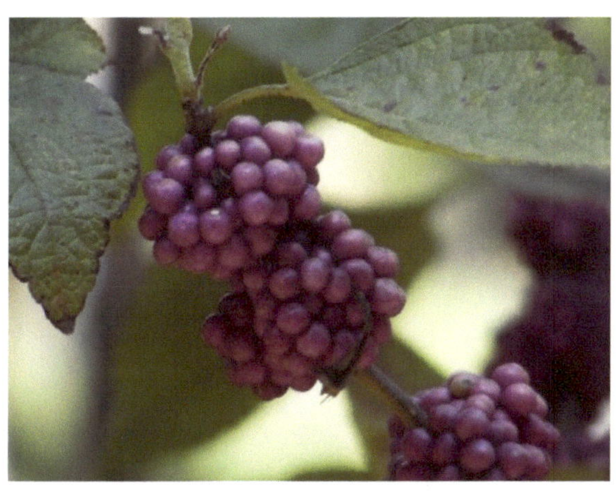

Enlighten Your Mind

Dear Lord, grant us Your Spirit of Peace and Love. Let Your Holy Spirit guide our life. Enlighten our mind and bestow upon us Holy Divine Light. We ask to enter Your Most Holy Presence. Guide and help us to receive Your Gift of inner peace and sacred silence. Lead us to awareness of Holy inspiration. Help us always to know that we are secure in the Hands of the Creator. There is a Divine purpose to fulfill. Be with us now and eternally to guide and protect. Inspire within us wisdom, understanding, and knowledge of Your Word. Bring blessings to all whom we know and love.

Reference

Stroh, Frances RN, MA, FCN. Abide in Love the Sacred Presence of God,
    Meditative Prayer for Spiritual Care. Tolcare Books, 2015.

Stroh, Frances RN, MA, FCN, Awakening to the Holy Light of Christ, Touch of
    Life Meditative Prayer for Inner Peace, Tolcare Books, 2014.

Stroh, Frances RN, MA, FCN. God Speaks in Peaceful Momemts of Prayer,
    Living in the Spirit of God, Tolcare Books, 2016.

Stroh, Frances RN, Ph.D., FCN. Healing Arts and Science to Alleviate Pain,
    Spiritual Care of Body, Mind, and Spirit, Tolcare Books, 2019.

Stroh, Frances RN, Ph.D., FCN. Journey in Divine Spirit, Gateway to Heavenly
    Peace, Tolcare Books, 2019.

Stroh, Frances RN, MA, FCN, Tracey Rzepka, MS, ARNP, FCN, Nancy Roberts,
    RN, CHPN, FCN, Beverly Granger, RN, FCN, Sue Nardy RN, FCN, P.J.
    May, RN, MSN, FCN, Bonnie Lanyi, RN, FCN. Tools for Health
    Ministry, God's Work Our Hands. Edited by RN, CHPN, FCN Nancy
    Roberts. Sarasota, Florida: Florida-Bahamas Synod Parish Nurse
    Network, 2011.

Stroh, Frances RN, MA, CH. Valley of the Silent Stream, Meditative Imagery
    for Iner Healing, Author House, Blumington, Indiana, 2006.

"Scripture quotations taken from the New American Standard
Bible® (NABS),Copyright © 1960, 1962, 1963, 1968, 1971, 1972, 1973, 1975,
1977, 1995. The Lockman Foundation. Used by permission. www.
Lockman.org"

About the Author

Frances Stroh RN, PhD., FCN, is a Faith Community Nurse, Auxiliary Ordained Interfaith Chaplain, Author, and Certified Clinical Hypnotherapist. She graduated from Queensborough Community College with a degree in Nursing Science in 1982. Then attended the University of the State of NY, Old Westbury, and Saint John's University, CA. She received a Bachelor of Science and Master of Arts Degree in Counseling Psychology and a Doctor of Philosophy, PhD., in Spiritual Healing.

Honors: Magna Cum Laude, and Honorary Doctor of Healing Arts and Sciences. Ongoing education in Community Health, Counseling Psychology, Wholistic Nursing, Therapeutic Touch, Biofeedback, Faith Community Nursing, and Clinical Hypnotherapy. Publications include seven books on meditative prayer for spiritual care. Experience includes, psychiatric, mental health, developmental disabilities, wholistic, faith community nursing, and school nursing.

Since 2009 Frances is a Faith Community Nurse at Our Savior Lutheran Church in Vero Beach Florida. Health and Eucharistic Minister, leader of Sisters in Christ Care, Healing prayer, and Meditation group. Also, pastoral care visitation, and leader of Spirituality Group at the Behavioral Health Center, Cleveland Clinic, Indian River Hospital in Vero Beach FL.